Resol...
Techniq... ... ...eau a Life without Pain

Resolving Pain provides an insightful exposé on understanding the cause and effect of back pain. Dr. Worrell also provides clear instructions for understanding and treating back pain. Through Dr. Worrell's methodologies, I have experienced significant relief for my own occasional back pain.
Arun Badi, MD, PhD
Board Certified ENT and Sleep Medicine Physician
Adjunct Professor, Department of Electrical and Computer Engineering
University of Texas, Dallas

It was a pleasure to read *Resolving Pain*. The principles and techniques described in the book are straightforward and easy to understand. I identified with much of this lovely and encouraging book. Dr. Worrell presents a natural approach to disengaging the self-protection mechanism and engaging inner peace to relax and heal the body. I know many people could benefit from Dr. Worrell's simple techniques for pain relief.
Jane Wells
Artist and Designer

Maricel Forteza

Please enjoy the
benefit of this

Paul S Worrell D

Resolving Pain

Proven Non-Surgical Techniques to Lead a Life without Pain

Paul Stephen Worrell, DO

Resolving Pain

www.resolvingpain.com

ISBN: 978-1-937045-04-3

Published by

Lovett Press International

214-350-1696

ann@lovettconsulting.com

For direct book orders or speaking engagements, contact:

Paul Stephen Worrell, DO

at

resolvingpain@gmail.com

Dedication

I dedicate this book to my wife Karen and to my children, Linda, Nathan, David, Paul II, Lauren, Adam, Katie, Julianne and Sean—in the hopes that future generations will not have to suffer from back pain.

Acknowledgments

I am so very grateful to my parents, John and Jo Worrell, for giving me life and always encouraging me to follow my calling and perform all of my work with excellence.

I am also deeply indebted to my dear and longtime friends, Laurie and Terry Pace for supporting me and encouraging me to write this book. Thanks to Laurie for building my website for this book.

Thank you to Nagaraj Kikkeri, MD, of the NTTC Surgery Center in Mesquite Texas for his contribution to this book regarding pain management and his continuing support of my quest to relieve patients' pain.

Thank you to my publisher, Ann Lovett Baird, and her team at Lovett Press International for their expertise and dedication to releasing this book.

Foreword

Resolving Pain gives clear and decisive information designed to inspire individuals to self-analyze their chronic pain. Dr. Worrell explains the use of biofeedback to help readers determine the source of pain, providing a holistic approach to improving their mindset toward pain, which is key to pain management. Rather than assuming that they have to live with pain or submit to surgery, readers are encouraged to disengage the body's self-protection mechanism to relieve chronic pain.

Dr. Worrell describes what pain is and breaks it down into digestible components, so that anyone can understand what causes pain and the body's response to it. He introduces the concept of pain patterns and the pain-guarding cycle, and also

Resolving Pain

explains that pain can be caused by stress, which

readers may not be aware of. He also provides

physical and mental techniques, and exercises to

help relieve pain, and shares vignettes of positive

results that his patients have experienced.

Well worth the read, Dr. Worrell brings new

light to relieving chronic pain in a holistic way. He

brings hope to all who suffer from chronic pain.

Nagaraj Kikkeri, MD
Board Certified Anesthesiologist, specializing in
pain medicine

NTTC Surgery Center
3865 Childress Ave,
Mesquite, TX 75150

TABLE OF CONTENTS

Introduction

Some of the most insightful thoughts and amazing stories, many of which could have helped people change their lives, were never actually written, spoken or shared. It was pure genius lost . . . like the ripples that subside and then disappear from the wake of a boat. What would our lives be like if some of these pearls of wisdom were actually written and pursued?

My decision to write this book was prompted by my own chronic back pain, which had been part of my life for ten years. My daily struggle with this level of pain made me empathetic toward other people who were suffering. As a Doctor of Osteopathic Medicine (DO), the challenge lay before me. I knew I had to figure out how to heal myself and then I could pursue teaching other medical professionals and individuals how to heal themselves. Writing this book started with my pain and my quest to stop it.

I like to take on things that are difficult and challenging. They may be easy for others, but my personal satisfaction is immense when I can do something well, especially when I was not even sure I could do it at all. Problems create opportunities for solutions. My chronic back pain was an opportunity. I lived with it for many years, just accepting that chronic back pain was going to be my way of life, until I knew I had to accept the challenge to find a solution.

My hope is this book will encourage you to look past your chronic pain to a future of no pain, a future where you actually feel healthy. I offer a plan that will keep your back pain or other acute or chronic pain from recurring.

Pain is caused by one of two reasons: physical damage or "guarding," which can also be called flinching. There is not a third reason why you have pain. This book is not about fixing physical damage, which may require surgery or other solutions. It's about stopping pain due to flinching, which in my experience is the most common source of chronic pain. Physical damage may need to be addressed by a different approach than I offer, and I give due respect to those who are successful with other approaches. The techniques I describe can be used on their own to bring complete relief or to supplement other kinds of treatment including physical therapy, chiropractic care, acupuncture or even surgery.

Although this approach is not going to offer everyone total relief, the majority of those who properly apply it will find, as I have, that it is beneficial, both as a physician and a sufferer of chronic pain. People who find the greatest relief are those who commit to repeatedly and consistently using these techniques for ongoing relief. Relief becomes a motivation, so that you continue with the techniques until your pain is gone.

It Started with My Pain

It was a bright, beautiful winter day in
Colorado. I was on a ski vacation with my children,
and in need of play and exercise, we decided to take
a race across the parking lot at our hotel. Before
reaching the other side, I slipped on the ice and
landed flat on my back. The fall on that hard, icy
concrete was so severe that it took several minutes
for me to catch my breath. When I fell, I heard what
sounded like crackers crumbling and felt a sharp
pain in my low back. I knew then I had injured
myself severely. Sure enough, I had—and for ten
years I had back pain every day.

Over those ten years, some days were worse
than others. I modified my life and physical
movements, attempting to live with the pain. I gave

5

little, if any thought to the reason why my back

hurt, because I assumed my pain was solely due to

the damage from the ice-related injury. People

would see me walking awkwardly and ask what was

wrong. I told them that I hurt my back from a fall

on the ice. They understood that. I, along with

anyone else I spoke to, seemed to accept the idea

that my accident caused my pain and there was

nothing I could do to change it. It made perfect

sense that the pain I felt and the way I moved was

expected. I never stopped to think that there might

be another reason why I was experiencing pain.

If I was lying down, I couldn't even sit up

without first rolling to my side and pushing up with

my hands. I remember trying to figure out the best

way to get up off the floor to avoid pain. I crawled

on my hands and knees to a chair to pull myself up,
and then used the nearby wall to get to a standing
position. Then, at least for a while, I could
cautiously walk with my bottom carefully tucked
under my back.

No one, including me, ever asked the
question, "Could it be that the injury was just the
start of the pain?"

To which I would have replied, "Do you not
understand how hard concrete under ice is?
Obviously, you have no idea how bad my back
feels!"

In retrospect, this was nothing more than
justification for my pain. What I saw as a clear
perception of my situation was nothing more than a
wrong assumption. I was so lost in my pain, I never

stopped to really consider that perhaps the injury was what initiated the pain, but it wasn't the sole cause. I never even considered that my body's reaction to pain could be prolonging or exacerbating the pain.

Ten years after my fall on the ice, I was at a conference with colleagues in San Diego instructing other doctors how to take care of neck and back pain for their patients, using Ligamentous Articular Strain techniques. These techniques are based on the 1940s work of William G. Sutherland, DO. We divided his writings into specific topics. During the conference, as I was preparing to teach, I realized that I really had nothing of consequence to say to these people if I was still hurting after ten years. What credibility did I have if I couldn't even fix my own pain? So I thought, "Okay physician, heal thyself."

Knowing that I had to give these physicians something useful to help them help others,   I started thinking about the idea that if I hurt my shoulder, I would hold it in a guarded fashion. Even if I didn't hurt my shoulder, and held it in a guarded fashion, it would hurt from holding it that way. Guarding yourself from additional pain is innate. Our bodies do it without us consciously thinking about it. So, if I was guarding my back from additional pain by holding it a certain way, that could actually cause additional pain, because my body was now reacting to the way I was guarding it. I thought about how I had been living in my body since I fell on the ice. The muscles in my back were so tight that I couldn't even walk upright.

I wondered whether my pain was due to the damage done falling on the ice, or from my body guarding me from additional pain?

If I were in pain due to guarding, how would I stop the cycle? I knew that if I could relax the tension in my back, perhaps it would stop hurting. So, I figured I could either release the tension by just "dropping it," or hold the muscles tight enough, long enough that they would fatigue, lose tension and relax.

So I tucked my tailbone under my back and squeezed my gluteus muscles as tight as I could until they fatigued, meaning I could literally not hold them tight anymore. I was astounded that my pain subsided. Then I felt it start to creep back, so I did it again, and the pain subsided. I repeated this process until I had no pain. I was amazed that after ten years of walking around all wadded up due to pain, it was now completely gone!

This was a monumental shift for me. I hadn't been thinking about how I could make my pain stop. I accepted that I fell on the ice and hurt my back, and that the ten years of pain was due to the damage done by the injury. Now I realized that while the initial injury caused excruciating pain, it impacted how I carried my body and ultimately made my pain worse.

I realized that pain comes from only two sources: damaged tissue or guarding the body against more pain. There isn't a third source of pain.

Resolving Pain

When I started using what I discovered about my own pain with my patients, I was able to show them how to relieve their bodies of pain. Using simple techniques, I found patients could relieve themselves of their chronic or acute pain.

Even though the pain from my fall and the ten years of suffering were not pleasant, if that had not happened to me, I might not have discovered the miraculous techniques that I learned and now use with my patients.

In this book I'll give you tools to problem solve and relieve your own pain. It takes diligence to relieve chronic pain, and I have plenty of patients who have found amazing relief using the techniques presented in this book.

What is Pain?

Pain is essentially a signal that something is wrong. Your body gives you pain to protect you from doing more damage. In some cases, it's a combination of tissue damage and your body reacting to that tissue damage to prevent more pain. If you have tissue damage that causes pain, then you may flinch, or guard, for fear of more pain. If you sprain, bruise or contuse your tissue, you'll be sore from that action, but when you flinch to protect yourself from more pain, it unfortunately just makes it worse.

People will come to me and say, "Doctor, it hurts when I do this."

Resolving Pain

And what do I tell them? "Then stop doing that!"

In a sense, your pain is telling you what your boundaries are. When you're driving down the highway and happen to veer out of your lane, you feel the rumble of the lane markers, which signals that you need to adjust and get back into your lane. Your pain is doing the same thing. It's telling you that you're out of a safe boundary and you need to stop doing what you're doing. You need to make a course correction with how you're moving or posturing your body.

Body Language

Your body has a language all its own that is predictable. Your body thinks pain means only one thing . . . that you're being attacked. The fact is, when your body feels threatened, you physically react without thinking about it. Your body reacting to pain as though you're being attacked is innate and predictable. In terms of involuntary responses like muscles tensing, everyone's body responds the same way. For instance, if someone swings his or her fist at your face, it's human nature to hold your hand up to protect your face, and specific muscles tense up. Some will respond more intensely than others, but that's really the only difference in how each person's body reacts.

Your brain has a built-in defense mechanism on a very fundamental level that causes your body to defend you from harm. Let's look at what happens when your flinch reflex comes into play.

Resolving Pain

When you flinch, the amygdala region of
your brain sends a distress signal so that the
hypothalamus activates the sympathetic nervous
system, sending signals through the autonomic
nerves to the adrenal glands. These glands respond
by pumping the hormone epinephrine, also known
as adrenaline, into the bloodstream. Adrenaline is
released in reaction to strong emotions like fear or
stress to help your body react more
quickly. It makes the heart beat faster, increases
blood flow to the brain and muscles, and
stimulates the body to make sugar to use for fuel.
Your body does not know if the pain is due to
flinching or tissue damage, so it takes any kind of
pain as a threat.

Pain Guarding Cycle

When the body processes pain as a threat it produces guarding or the flinch reflex. This creates a cycle that is hard to break. Many medical professionals will call this a *pain spasm cycle*. The problem with the word *spasm* is that it indicates that you cannot control or re-train the cycle.

Your self-protection mechanism is something you can reprogram. It is not an external force that you have no control over. This cycle is better termed the *pain guarding cycle*. Once that pain communication and flinch reflex is established, the brain is working against you, by keeping that cycle going. This is why it can be very hard for my patients to stop the action they say causes their pain, even when I'm telling them this can solve the problem. The brain refuses to alter its pattern. The pain, as well as the fear of pain, prompts the brain's pattern, or self-protection mechanism. You may also get emotionally involved with your pain by getting angry, scared or frustrated. This only keeps the cycle going.

Pain from Stress

Pain is not just a by-product of physical injury. It can manifest itself through increased daily stress and your predictable response to that stress. For example, if you have a confrontation with a co-worker your shoulders may tense up. You get a call from a loved one who sternly says, "We need to talk, but we'll do it when you get home." What happens? The same thing: your shoulders tense up. Now holding that stress in your shoulders causes altered posture. It's predictable that you respond to stress by holding it in your shoulders. Other people might respond to stress in different ways. No matter how you hold the stress, it's going to cause you to pain. Your body says, "Oh, it's a threat!" and the cycle continues.

In this way, we are like turtles. When we feel attacked, we draw our limbs into our shell for protection. The only problem is that we don't have a shell, so pulling our limbs in provides no protection, and we wind up wadding up our bodies and exacerbating our pain.

Summary

Realizing that pain is nothing more than information prompting a physical response is the first step to figuring out its origin. In a sense, pain is your friend. It's trying to tell you to adjust the way you hold yourself in the face of injury or even a stressful day.

Pain is helpful because it tells you that something is wrong. Pain can originate from physical injury, then morph into long-term pain if you automatically react to the pain or fear of more pain. Your body has a built-in self-protection mechanism that interprets pain as an attack. It cannot tell the difference between pain from injury versus pain from flinching. It treats all pain as though it is an attack, which starts a *pain guarding cycle*.

In some cases, pain originates from emotions like stress, anger, frustration or resentment. Your physical reaction to an emotional situation can cause you to tense up and react in a way that will cause immediate or even chronic pain.

The notion of a *pain spasm cycle* espoused by medical professionals indicates you have no control over your pain or stopping it. This implies that you're a victim unable to solve the problem. You're not a victim. In the next chapter, we'll look at how to solve the problem.

Resolving Pain

Solving the Problem

How you choose to approach a problem directly impacts whether you'll be able to solve it. You begin with what you think are the facts, then you assume that if there's a solution it will be based on the understanding that the facts are correct. Depending on your approach, you're either working as a problem solver or as a victim. The most you can hope for as a victim is pity. As a problem solver, you can move in the direction of finding a solution. You play one role or the other.

All of us are guilty of making wrong assumptions. For certain, I was wrong to blame my back pain solely on my injury from falling on the ice. For ten years I fully embraced this belief and I paid for that with chronic back pain. I feel fortunate that my pain is gone, and to this day, more than twenty years later, I have not suffered any more pain related to my fall.

In order to find success with the techniques that I present in this book, you first need to recognize that the problem may be due to something other than the initial injury. Knowing that there's a possible solution to the problem can motivate you to pursue it. Second, you and your health care provider need a clear understanding of what the problem truly is. You can't solve the problem if you don't understand it. Third, you need to give a complete and dedicated effort to the techniques I present in this book in order to see results. Since you're reprogramming your self-protection mechanism, you have to work diligently to disengage it. And, if you do something that hurts, that self-protection mechanism will re-engage.

As a problem solver, you have to teach yourself to live differently in your body. It's not something you'll necessarily do overnight.

Figuring it Out

The diagnostic technique I discovered that day at the conference in San Diego is what I call flinch analysis. Your body has a predictable response to a threat, no matter who you are. In this regard, everyone's body is programmed the same. If someone comes at your shoulder with a weapon, you can predict that your reflex is dodging, and muscle contractions. As I mentioned earlier, the only difference in the way people react is the intensity. Intensity is affected by certain personality traits and how physically strong you are.

Physical Damage Versus Flinching

Since we know that pain comes from only two sources: physical tissue damage or flinching, we can use that definitive information to understand the source of the problem.

So, to figure out how to relieve someone of pain we have to figure out how much of it is coming from tissue damage and how much is coming from flinching. While there are many places on the body that can help you determine this, we will focus on two key pressure points on your body in this book. If the pain is coming from flinching, these particular spots will be abnormally tender.

Pressure Points

You can use these pressure points any time you have pain to determine whether you're flinching.

First, there is a pressure point on the back of your hand, between the last knuckle of your thumb and your wrist. You can use your other hand to find that spot by applying pressure to determine whether you are flinching. This technique is described in more detail later in this book.

The second is the piriformis muscle, which is on the outside of the bone you sit on. If you apply pressure to this muscle and it's tender, that's an indicator that you're flinching—most likely in your neck or back.

Resolving Pain

Biofeedback

If you find that spot on your hand is more
tender than normal, allow your shoulders and chest
to relax as you breathe out. When the flinch has
been released from your shoulder or neck, you'll
notice that the pain in your hand goes away. This is
known as biofeedback. It's a wonderful way to
remind yourself not to wear your stress, or let
physical pain change your natural posture, which
will cause more pain. Now you have a tool to help
you relieve your pain—anytime, anywhere.

The other pressure point you can use for
biofeedback techniques is your piriformis muscle. If
you sit on a wadded-up sock on your piriformis and
it's tender, then release tension from the place in
your body that is hurting. You are *not* trying to

massage pain out by rubbing against the sock, only determine if your self-protection mechanism is engaged. When your piriformis is no longer tender, you know you have tamed the flinch reflex for the time being.

Some patients will try using a tennis ball against their piriformis, then, come back to the office and say that sitting on or rubbing against the tennis ball did not work. In some cases, they have actually reengaged the self-protection mechanism because the body thinks the pain of the pressure from the tennis ball is an attack.

As I have said before, if what you are doing creates pain, then stop what you're doing. The pain will only reengage the self-protection mechanism, prolonging your pain cycle.

Self-Protection Mechanism

The fact that the built-in self-protection mechanism cannot distinguish between pain from injury versus pain from flinching can foster the pain cycle. However, this built-in primitive response has value. For instance, when you touch something hot, your natural reaction of pulling your hand away saves you from getting burned. When attacked, this self-protection mechanism stimulates a reflex response. As the car door is about to close on your fingers, you instinctively pull them away. You don't think about it, you just do it. I cannot emphasize this enough. Your pain creates a context for more pain because of the self-protection mechanism. In a sense, the mechanism feeds on your chronic pain.

There is nothing profound about what I am describing here. Virtually everyone understands a predictable response to pain, but I want to point out how easily you can anticipate the body's response to pain or even the threat of pain or injury. Anyone can predict what the response would be if you put someone against the wall and poked them. Depending on where you poke them, and how hard you poke them, you could accurately predict their response because everyone's muscles tense the same way to the same type of attack.

Be Observant

If you closely analyze the flinching response to pain, details of the pattern emerge. If you hurt your shoulder, it is not your shoulder that responds, it is that entire side of your body. You can see the

31

energy pattern in the tensing of muscles. Muscle tension causes tenderness in those muscles. Recognizing this tenderness was the basis for developing Shiatsu or acupressure.

You don't wad yourself up, for the most part, as an intentional effort to hurt yourself. The built-in self-protection mechanism is there to protect you from danger. Unfortunately, it can work against you. The *fear* of more pain causes you to flinch, which intensifies the pain and causes it to linger.

Once you know the root cause of your flinch response from careful observation of what your body is telling you, you can begin to solve the problem. You'll find that simply asking yourself

why you're hurting will help you stop doing the
action that's hurting you.

A critical point: if it hurts don't do it. If pain
intensifies, it will keep you from getting better. You
may feel like you have to work through pain. The
fact is, when you try to work through pain, your
self-protection mechanism is engaged, trying you to
save you from more pain.

Early Intervention

There's a tendency for pain to become
habitual. It's like that bad habit that you can't seem
to stop doing, even though you know you should.
Bad habits are hard to break because the brain likes
to repeat things. It looks for repeated patterns. The
longer you have a habit, the harder it is to break.
Early intervention, by disrupting the body's innate

response to pain, lessens the complexities and effort required to dismantle this response.

You may experience an emotional overlay that becomes a complication if you feel victimized by the pain. You may get angry, frustrated, depressed or lose sleep as a result of your pain. Once emotion comes into play, you may feel tormented. If you feel victimized by pain, it's hard to turn back. By nature, victims are not good problem solvers. Confidence in your ability to solve problems empowers you. It encourages creative thinking and inspires you to make the effort required to find success.

Isometrics

While biofeedback helps you determine that the self-protection mechanism is impacting your pain and helps you release that pain, isometrics is a method that helps you release tension and tightness in muscles. With isometrics you hold a muscle tight enough, long enough in order to wear it out. This is called muscle failure. When you cannot hold the muscle tight anymore, you have muscle failure and you get relief from pain.

When taking the muscles to failure, you cannot quit when you're tired, you have to continue until the muscle has lost its tension. A warning: If something you're doing hurts or produces worse than minor discomfort, stop right away.

Simple Solution

Everything in life can be simplified. All the information and music ever recorded can be converted to 0s or 1s, which is the same binary language of computers. The approach presented here is truly very simple. As I mentioned earlier, pain comes for two reasons:

- Injury: When you're damaged, you hurt. If you're torn, broken, contused or have arthritis, you're going to have pain.

- Flinching: Whenever you feel pain for any reason, you experience a predictable response. If you're sitting at a stoplight and you see a car coming in your rearview mirror that you know can't stop in time to avoid hitting you, your body tenses, bracing for the collision. Your injuries from the car accident are exacerbated by the fact that your body was tense at the point of impact. Then you may walk around tense, trying not

to magnify your injuries from the car
accident and avoid more pain, which just
makes matters worse.

When pressure points are tender to touch
representing a flinch, you have two options:

- Biofeedback to tell your body to drop the
  pain.

- Isometrics, to hold the muscle tight enough,
  to achieve muscle failure.

Resolving Pain

Summary

To problem-solve your pain, recognize it's likely that your pain is due to flinching. As much as ninety percent of most muscle pain is from flinching.

You and your health care provider need a clear understanding of specific areas of tenderness that almost always indicate that the flinch is operating. Flinch analysis can rule out pain from injury. Injury is not necessarily the default reason for your pain.

For the techniques described in this book to work, you need to devote concerted and continuous effort toward relieving your pain. Anything less than an all-out effort will yield little, if any, results.

You have to use the techniques on an ongoing basis to keep your pain away.

Use biofeedback from the tender spot in your hand or piriformis to identify and release pain from a specific location in your body. All pain comes from tissue injury or the flinch response. The flinch response can be a result of your initial injury, fear of future injury or emotional factors like stress. Keen observation of what your body is telling you is key to solving your pain problem. Early intervention in your pain cycle will make stopping the pain easier.

Resolving Pain

Stopping the Pain

Back to Basics

Obviously, the best way to avoid back or any other type of chronic pain is not to set yourself up for it. Don't get hurt or injured, don't engage in activities that cause damage, don't be born with genetics that cause arthritis, don't eat foods that cause joints to hurt, don't be overweight, or don't get stressed. Easy, right? But you don't live in a bubble. Things happen, and your genetics were put into place long before you were born. So, avoiding pain by dealing with some of the above issues could be a start, but not every factor at play is under your control.

Overall, I'd generalize that ninety percent of the pain my patients typically experience is due to the self-protection mechanism and ten percent is due to tissue damage. While tissue damage may have caused the initial pain, the self-protection mechanism kept it going.

Strong Challenge

Competitive, strong-spirited or physically stronger people have to work harder than others to get their body to break down the built-in self-protection mechanism.

Physically strong people may be dissuaded from putting out the effort it takes to reach muscle failure because they're so strong their muscles are very tight in the first place. They stop before they realize the value of the effort.

And truly, I've found strong spirited people are more likely to have back problems. Why?

Because there's something built into them that's naturally competitive. These people are more intense and wound more tightly than others. In some cases, they are rebellious in the sense that they don't want to be told what to do. That rebelliousness can also prevent them from thinking positively, which is what they have to do in order to alleviate pain. They must believe that the techniques and exercises will work. If someone can't look ahead to feeling better, focusing on dreams of a pain-free future or living in their bodies differently becomes a challenge. If someone cannot focus on the future, they start to focus on the pain. The result is a pity party and more pain.

Often, people who are strong spirited are also physically strong, which creates a double challenge. I don't say these things to be discouraging, only to say that people with these traits have to stick with it! They have to persevere while staying relaxed and calm, which can be difficult for people with strong wills or physically strong bodies. Constant and ongoing biofeedback is important in order to get relief. I have some patients who might go meditate to feel relaxed, but when they are done, they go back to their wadded-up tense selves. Using these techniques sometimes requires a change in lifestyle or mindset.

The fact is these techniques require relaxation and letting go. A tense mindset will work against someone. They cannot *make* themselves relax, which is the mindset they use to accomplish most other things. They have to *allow* themselves to relax.

There is no sense in dwelling on what cannot be changed. Often, you may be left with how to make the best of a bad situation. The good news is that you do have options. How you respond to injury or disease has much to do with how much pain you actually experience. Let's focus on what you can change. This does not mean living in denial, but instead, looking toward a future with no pain. You have to be aggressively optimistic because the absence of this will lead to despair.

What do You Believe?

If you believe that the pain you have is totally due to physical damage, you're severely limiting your approach to dealing with it. If you

45

believe X-rays, CAT scans and MRIs are the only

way to analyze the source of pain, you may be

missing an opportunity to get better or even totally

stopping the pain. It's so easy to take on a victim

mentality as a physician points to damage on

images. Well-meaning physicians are guided by

studying these images, but their approach is related

to the mechanics of injury, or an issue related to

anatomical changes. Orthopedic surgeons look for a

solution using surgery because that is what they're

trained for. That's what they know how to do.

On numerous occasions people have come

to my office, explaining that their back pain is due

to bulging discs. Knowing that all of us in time can

get bulging discs and degenerative changes in the

back, I explain to people that their diagnostic

images do not necessarily warrant surgical intervention, nor do they show the cause of the person's pain. The vast majority of CAT scans and MRIs do not offer evidence that surgery is warranted, and in these cases, I encourage people not to jump to that option right away. The techniques for disarming the self-protection mechanism can provide relief without surgery. It's worth the time to given them a try before going under the knife. After all, there are no guarantees that surgery will eliminate the pain.

Medical images are valuable pieces of the puzzle when you're looking at surgical options. However, if you're not sure about or willing to submit to surgery, there is questionable value in doing expansive study of images to determine surgical options.

I see myself as a problem-solver, and most of the people who come to me for help with their back pain find relief. There is a strong possibility that these techniques will work for you too, and you can experience a significant reduction or elimination of pain.

For some, disengaging the self-protection mechanism works, and that's all that they need. For others, disengaging the self-protection mechanism serves as a supplement to other treatment. A combination of physical therapy, various forms of manipulation, Pilates, yoga, acupuncture, and even surgery can work together to give people relief.

Manipulation frees up what got stuck from muscle tension. I like to do manipulation after assisting the patient with isometrics to the point of muscle failure. This is not the type of manipulation that can cause damage. If someone has pain from vertebrae getting stuck, they have to get unstuck first, in order to disengage the self-protection mechanism. However, I might have to use isometrics to get muscles to relax before I can use manipulation to get them unstuck.

Hope

In order to help anyone, they must first believe there is hope. Without hope, the patient might ask, "Why should I ever try something that might help if help is not possible?"

Resolving Pain

They might just ask for pain medicine and muscle relaxers and hope to live with it. People who work with sincere effort are more likely to find success. For these techniques to work, the person has to be committed and go the distance.

Having done this for many years, I can predict with fair accuracy, who will do well with my approach. Those who are sincere about getting help and have a healthy work ethic are the best candidates. This type of patient understands the concept and is willing to do whatever it takes to stop the pain. Essentially you have to change the way you live in your body. People who don't believe the techniques will work or approach it with sarcasm typically will not succeed.

You must first recognize that the inappropriate tension in the muscles is a response to initial pain, with tenderness as the indicator. It's like you're taking layers of tension off, giving the body a temporary reprieve, then repeating the exercise.

So how can a technique that offers only temporary results offer any hope for long-term relief? The techniques retrain your self-protection mechanism, which takes time. Think of world-class athletes. They didn't get that way overnight. Many years of training and practice got them to their level of skill and ability.

Personally, I have been fortunate enough to go more than twenty years without back pain. If I can do it, you can too! Vigilance and repetition are the keys. If you are tense but don't know it, you are

51

not excused from the pain that comes from being all wadded up. You cannot address problems you don't see. Fortunately, you can recognize flinch patterns based on tenderness at the two pressure points I described earlier.

Mindset

Are you tired of hurting? Have you hurt badly enough, long enough to do what it takes to quit hurting? Are you willing to look at a different approach and put in enough effort to change your approach to life? Do you believe it's possible to reprogram your innate, built-in self-protection mechanism? If your approach to finding relief needs a boost or if you want to try something new to help, this may be what you're looking for. You have to have the mindset that you're in control of your body and a great problem solver.

If you believe there is a good reason why you should choose to do what feels good rather than what causes you to hurt, you're less likely to stray into pain. If you're an optimist with hope and joy, you're going to be more relaxed. If you're a pessimist living with sadness and fear, this leaves you all wadded up and tense. If you truly have faith, what reason do you have for wearing fear? For that matter, what other excuses do you have for being tense?

Your mindset cannot let influences from the outside impact your stress level. No one else has control of you. You have a choice in how you react to situations. If someone yells at you, you have a natural defense mechanism that wants to protect you. You may withdraw inside yourself, get stressed or lash out at the person. If you're at peace with yourself, you can figure that the problem lies with the person yelling, not with you. If you speak peacefully back to the person, they might actually calm down.

When you have an attitude of gratitude, it shapes the way you view things. When you think "what a pleasure to have this opportunity," you're less likely to ponder what you like, hate or resent about a task. Aligning your thoughts with appreciation will give you a better outlook on life and can actually help relieve your pain.

You give power to whatever thoughts you focus on. If you focus on the fact that there are good reasons for your pain, you'll slip into the trap of justification. If you think there are good reasons for your anger, stress or pain, you'll stay stuck there.

My goal for you and all of my patients is to have a pain-free life. It is truly about feeling good. For you, pain may be nothing more than a symptom of a failed approach. As you know, the flinch is a necessary means of self-protection. When the door is about to slam on your finger, you quickly withdraw it without thinking. You pull your hand from the hot pot to avoid being burned.

My point is that your intent to live with appreciation and goals tends to keep you pointed in the right direction as you drive down the road of life. If you subscribe to the right philosophy at the start of physical damage done, you can limit your

Resolving Pain

pain by monitoring and turning off the self-protection mechanism. As an example, a bulging disc has the force of gravity and the weight of the person's body resting atop the damaged zone. Then the tensing of the muscles between the vertebrae exacerbates the pain. Early intervention can get you closer to a positive frame of mind more quickly. The sooner you do something to retrain the flinch from a bulging disc, the more likely you'll get relief.

Peace of Mind

Focusing on your peace of mind keeps you from focusing on your pain. You don't *work* to have peace of mind; you *accept* it as a gift. Inner peace ensures that you're less focused on the pain or fear of it, so your body feels less need to protect you from pain. You can work toward peace of mind in many ways. Various religions, meditation and self-hypnosis offer a format to bring about change. You have to continually monitor yourself to validate that you're *wearing* inner peace.

Peace of mind requires some forethought, but it's also easy to overthink, which can move you away from experiencing serenity in the body. It's almost like you have to get a little stupid to find peace.

So often I have seen people work so hard to manipulate themselves into relaxing. *Over thinkers will* try to *think* themselves into relaxing by "taking charge" and try to force themselves to a relaxed position. People who live in fear or anger may empower those feelings to the point where they just don't know how to relax. Feeling justified in those feelings leads them to victim behavior, which says they *can't* relax. The root of the problem can be that they have no peace of mind, meaning they have no way to get comfortable inside their bodies. The negative thinking keeps them stuck in a feeling pattern that prevents them from having inner peace. To be clear, what I focus on with patients is whether they hurt and how much, but peace of mind can play a big role in pain.

Everyone seems to have limits regarding how much pain they can tolerate. During the first fifteen years of my practice, I delivered 1,000 babies. Some women delivered naturally, and I watched how they handled the pain. So often, I witnessed that early in labor they would keep their focus. As the contractions got more intense, their eyes would dart, the neck and shoulders would flinch, then, they would clinch their fists more tightly. At this point, the woman might scream. There's no dignity in pain. I could tell these women to relax but at some point, they would grow impatient with the pain and ask for medication. Some patients kept focus during the birthing process and seemed to have less pain. They appeared to flow with the pain, rather than become impatient with it and tense up to fight it. I believe they suffered less because they were able to maintain focus and find peace of mind within the pain.

No one wants to hurt, but few people hold themselves accountable for getting comfortable in their own skin. In a way, people can think of reasons that predispose them to the pain. They find reasons for the pain, like:

"Something is wrong with my back."

"I strained my back."

"I fell and injured by back."

"My job stresses me out."

People blame something for the initial pain, then give it credit for ongoing pain, pain that's actually due to the flinch reflex. Often the person might have avoided injury in the first place if they had embraced finding a way to create peace of mind.

As an illustration, think of how you might create a hula-hoop. You would start with plastic tubing that you could bend into an arch, gluing the

ends together to form a circle. If you threaded the

tubing through a segment of pipe and tried to bend

it, it would kink at the end of the pipe segment. This

is similar to how most people pull their backs.

You're built so that you have flexibility to

bend at your hip joint and at the lumbosacral joint in

your lower back. When you have too much tension

in your buttocks, whatever the reason, when you

bend over you kink at the end of the pipe segment.

The tension in the gluteus piriformis region keeps

you from being able to bend at the hip. The fact that

the gluteus piriformis region is tight causes all the

flex when you are trying to bend over only at the

lumbosacral junction at the waist. This is not how

your body is designed to work, so you experience pain, or a pull in your back.

If you hurt your back that way, you might think everything was fine prior to bending over to picking up something. Actually, it was most likely due to tension in your buttocks that set you up for back injury. If you realized your buttocks were too tight and *turned off* the excess tension in those muscles prior to bending over, swinging a golf club or a tennis racket, you could have avoided the injury in the first place. As a golfer, tennis player or racquetball player, if you relieve tension in the buttocks prior to swinging, you're less likely to kink up and injure your back.

The interplay between lacking peace of mind and tight and tender muscles is like the thorn in your side — A person will continually tense up because of a failed approach to finding peace of mind. Often, they're just trying too hard or thinking too hard about having peace of mind. Then the person hurts because they're wadded up, which causes them to stress over the pain, then flinch harder, and so it goes . . .

Treatment

The healing arts, which encompasses many different approaches and methodologies, focuses on applying or developing techniques to help people use the body's systems to heal. New approaches are typically abandoned if they're not successful. Healing arts professionals do the best they can with the tools available. No matter what is being treated,

Resolving Pain

he or she will use tools based on how they were trained.

At times physical therapy, massages, acupuncture, medications, injections, nerve stimulation and manipulation treatments can provide temporary relief. There's simply not one approach that works for everyone. Some of these approaches are described below.

Physical Therapy

A physical therapist deals with the cycle of pain and guarding by using various approaches to induce a healing response. This includes conditioning, increasing strength and range of motion and improving transitions from one physical position to another in a way that doesn't cause pain.

Chiropractic Therapy

A chiropractor uses hands-on spinal manipulation to align the musculoskeletal structure. They also use manipulation techniques to restore mobility to joints restricted by tissue injury, which was caused by a traumatic event like falling.

Fitness Trainer Techniques

I use some of the same techniques a fitness trainer uses to motivate patients to take authority over their built-in self-protection mechanism. It's a tall order to break the body's instinctive need to save itself from pain without provoking the self-protection mechanism. It can be a vicious cycle. If it were not possible to dismantle the mechanism, I would still be in pain from my old injury, and I would not have had a good solution for so many

people who suffer from chronic pain.

Intervention Pain Management

A pain management specialist can formulate

a plan for interventional pain management

whenever there is a discernible and specific cause

for pain that is treatable. The pain management

specialist needs to develop a pain management plan

that is suited for a patient's specific situation. The

techniques described below can be used to ensure

surgical intervention is successful or prevent

unnecessary surgical interventions altogether. Not

all of these treatments are suitable for every patient.

Various modalities are used for injection

treatment, depending on the area of the body that is

impacted, such as neck also known as the cervical

spine, mid-back also known as the thoracic spine,
and the lower back known as the lumbar spine.
After careful evaluation by an interventional pain
specialist, these treatments are typically performed
at a pain management center in an operating room
setting. The interventional pain specialist uses either
a portable live x-ray called a fluoroscopy or
ultrasound machine.

Some of the most common interventional
treatments are the epidural steroid injection for low
back or leg pain, sacroiliac joint injection used to
treat lower back pain and/or sciatica symptoms, and
lumbar facet or medial branch blocks. A facet
block is an injection of local anesthetic and steroid
into a joint in the spine. A medial branch block is
similar, but the medication is placed outside the

joint space near the nerve that supplies the joint

called the medial branch. Sometimes pain

specialists use a selective nerve root block, which is

an injection of a long-lasting steroid around

the nerve root as it exits the spinal column. The

injection reduces the inflammation and pain caused

by pressure on the nerve.

Other interventional treatment modalities

include radio frequency rhizotomy that uses radio

frequency vibration to generate heat to the nerve

that is causing the pain. This essentially disrupts the

transmission of pain signals to the brain.

Spinal cord stimulation (SCS) is a therapy

that modulates pain signals before they reach the

brain. A small device, similar to a pacemaker, is

implanted in the body to deliver electrical pulses to

the spinal cord. It helps people better manage their chronic pain symptoms.

A pain pump using Intrathecal (IT) drug delivery system can relieve intractable pain. The system consists of an implantable pump that stores and delivers medication through a catheter to the IT space.

For more complex pain involving a compression fracture, technicians use kyphoplasty where a balloon is inserted into the fractured vertebrae space. After inflating the balloon and creating a space, acrylic bone cement is injected into the fractured area with live x-ray.

The overall goal of the interventional treatment is to assist and aid the patient in recuperating without major surgical intervention, if

possible.

Educating the Patient

To build a patient's belief and hope that I

can help them, often I encourage them to look at

their pain differently. If they believe all pain is

related to tissue damage, I need to help them

understand that tissue damage is not the only source

of pain. Typically, I'll begin with the shoulder pain

illustration:

I position myself like I'm having shoulder

pain and say, "If I hurt my shoulder, I would hold it

like this."

The patient nods.

"If nothing were wrong with my shoulder, but I held it that way, it would eventually hurt. If something you do hurts, I'll tell you to stop. There's no pain without a predictable response of guarding. That's the way your body is wired. You don't even think about it. The self-protection mechanism keeps the pain going in a vicious cycle. The body has its own communication method or body language."

I also explain to patients that the word *spasm* indicates there is no potential for stopping the pain. If someone holds on to the notion that they're having uncontrollable spasms, they essentially make themselves victims. The word *guarding* implies that someone has a choice. They choose to guard or not. For problem solvers, pain offers an opportunity to find a solution. They can turn off the pain caused by the tension in their muscles and the way they carry themselves. People should only have to suffer from the pain caused by injury, not the elongated cycle of pain from guarding or flinching.

I don't mind patients getting sore muscles or feeling briefly unstable from weakness after applying themselves, but if people hurt themselves trying to fatigue muscles, they only make the pain worse. It's like taking a stick to poke at a wild animal to tame it. Don't provoke your self-protection mechanism. I've said before, but I'm saying it again: if it hurts, don't do it.

Whether working with this approach or doing something else, do not do anything that causes pain, especially severe pain.

This is not unlike breaking a horse that runs in the front of the pack. If the horse trainer tries to *make* the horse follow commands, it will rebel. Using techniques to gain the horse's trust are much more effective. Forcing the horse to do what you want is like provoking the self-protection mechanism. It starts to work against you.

Physical Pain Creates Stress

The interplay between body language and the pain it causes leads to not only physical pain, but also emotional torment. How you feel about yourself impacts posture, speech pattern and thinking processes. You actually wear your desperation, anger, frustration or resentment if you feel like you're a victim of your pain. Then, as you wear these emotions, the body's reaction of increased muscle tension causes further pain and stress and predisposes you to other illnesses.

Many years ago, I had an aquarium. I noticed that when someone bothered or stressed the fish by tapping or slapping on the glass, the fish would get *tail rot* or *ick*. In the same way, when people get stressed, illness or disease follows. People may tend to blame outside stresses as the primary source, but it's the internal, indigenous stresses that hurt us the most.

Consistency

Although you need a basic plan directed toward the goal of finding peace with your body, you'll always have bumps in the road. You can't argue about how to deal with a certain set of issues and simultaneously be totally consumed with finding peace of mind. Being proactive about alleviating pain will work a lot better than being reactive.

In order for anyone to find hope in this technique, they have to see results. Some people will not put out the effort or underestimate what is required to break the spirit of the self-protection mechanism. Others, with effective coaching and motivational talk, will find temporary relief, only to later fall back into bad habits. If someone is inspired enough to find peace of mind and falls in love with that feeling and is motivated enough to do what they can to avoid pain, they will find the relief they seek.

Minimal effort typically gives minimal, if any response. If you can strip the body of its ability to save itself from pain, you can clearly see the value of this approach. It's so easy to become convinced that all the pain is from injury. Pain is never totally from injury. There is always a flinch component. When patients work hard enough to see the value, even temporarily, they're encouraged to believe that maybe there is hope. How else could it be that fatiguing muscles would offer any relief?

Summary

Stopping pain starts with believing it's possible not to hurt. Many times, patients come in with images from MRIs or X-rays that they feel prove they're going to be in pain. But oftentimes the images don't point to surgery. If the patient consistently applies techniques to turn off the self-protection mechanism, he or she will typically find relief.

Stress can cause pain as well. People with the tendency to get stressed about situations may find it more difficult to relax and stop the vicious cycle of stress, pain, flinch and more pain. This person may actually try or think too hard to achieve inner peace, which is something to be accepted as a gift. Peace of mind is the key to a long-term, pain-free life. People who focus on inner peace may

avoid getting injured in the first place.

Techniques

As you have probably surmised by reading this book, relaxing your muscles is the key to making these techniques work, which we'll explore in more depth in this chapter. To this point we have talked a lot about back pain, but the techniques I use can be employed to ease other types of pain. Please note that these exercises may not immediately release the pain. Your body has to work out the lactic acid that has built up over time. However, most of the time the results are immediate, within 10-15 minutes, especially for plantar fasciitis and knee pain.

Some of these techniques you can do by yourself. Others require two people. Please note that if what you're doing is causing pain, STOP

IMMEDIATELY. Not only could you be doing further tissue damage, you're re-engaging the self-protection mechanism any time you have pain. This is not a time to tough it out and work through your pain.

Self-Protection Mechanism Monitoring

As I've mentioned, your body has an automatic self-protection mechanism that causes you to flinch in order to guard you from pain. While there are a number of pressure points on your body to indicate whether the self-protection mechanism is engaged, there are two key pressure points I recommend exploring.

Hand Pressure Point Assessment

Find the spot on the back of your hand between the last knuckle of your thumb and your wrist. Use your other hand to find this pressure

point by applying pressure with your thumb. In

Exhibit 1 below, notice where the thumb from one

hand is applying pressure to the other. The black dot

near the thumb is another location where you can

apply pressure. Exhibit 2 shows the two locations

you can use on the hand as pressure points.

Exhibit 1

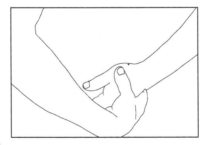

Exhibit 2

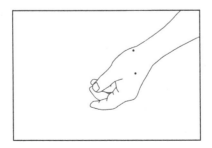

Resolving Pain

Don't press too hard, as you're only trying to monitor whether the self-protection mechanism is engaged. If you press on that pressure point just enough to feel tenderness, you know the self-protection mechanism is engaged. Then, you can drop it by relaxing your shoulders as you breathe out and you should notice that the pain in your hand goes away. This is known as biofeedback.

Piriformis Pressure Point Assessment

In order to locate the tender spot on your piriformis, which is outside of the bone you sit on, take a sock, wad it and drape yourself, half-lounged over the sock, so that it's under your piriformis. The dot in the diagram in Exhibit 3 indicates where your piriformis is located.

Exhibit 3

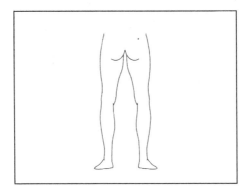

If you experience excruciating pain when you put your weight on the piriformis STOP doing the exercise and find something softer. This will determine if your leg is being pulled inside your torso, which can only be tender from guarding. If you sit on the sock and it's tender, find the place in your body where you're tense. Hold the tense muscle tight enough and long enough until you achieve muscle failure, meaning you can't hold it tight anymore. This is longer than just getting tired.

Resolving Pain

To really relieve the tension in the muscle, you have to wear it out.

If you have pain in your lower back, you can use this technique to find out how much of that pain is due to flinching. If the tender spot on the piriformis goes away, then you know you have released the flinch response. You're *not* trying to massage pain out by rubbing against the sock, you're only trying to determine if your self-protection mechanism is engaged. If you use something that's too hard, like a tennis ball, you could make your pain worse. The cardinal rule in stopping pain from flinching: don't do anything that causes excruciating pain. If you cause yourself more pain, you'll never break the cycle.

Pain Relief Exercises

In the pages that follow, I have described some exercises you can do to relieve pain in different parts of your body. Please remember that if anything increases your pain, stop immediately.

Shoulders

Start by monitoring your hand at the pressure point. If you find the self-protection mechanism is engaged, then you can use the following to get relief.

Get as comfortable as you can. Take a deep breath and let it out. Feel your chest collapse. Take another deep breath. Blow it out. Feel your shoulders drop. Let your shoulders feel like they're dropping all the way to the floor. Do this repeatedly so it becomes a way of carrying your shoulders.

Resolving Pain

You must learn to live in your body differently. At first, you may have to do this hundreds of times a day until you retrain yourself.

As I mentioned earlier, if you go around with all your muscles tense and poor posture to avoid pain, you're going to hurt from that. This relaxation technique is aimed at dismantling your self-protection mechanism. Predictably, the thing you fear if you're trying to relax your shoulders is fear of more pain in the shoulder. So repeatedly allowing your shoulders to relax will break that cycle. You need to make this a conscious and continuous effort, because the minute your shoulder starts to hurt a little bit, the self-protection mechanism will reengage. To be successful you must be proactive rather than reactive.

Upper Back

Your back hurts the way it does in the place it does because you're holding it too tight. Your pain is the guide. You have to think of your body as a system. Your upper back is connected to other parts of your body. These techniques work because pain often isn't just localized, it's caused because of another part of your body that's tight. Two ways you can deal with pain points in your upper back are listed below. Note that fatiguing the muscles can relieve the pain in another part of your body. If your back hurts, it can be due to your buttocks muscles being too tight. Fatiguing them will give the other part of your body that hurts relief.

Resolving Pain

Relax and Release Pain

Relax the place that is sore. Allow it to "drop out." Breathe deeply and imagine that the pain is leaving your body when you exhale.

Fatigue the Muscles

- Hold the muscle tight enough and long enough to fully fatigue it. To fully fatigue the muscle, you literally will not be able to hold it tight any longer. To get to this point, you may feel like your leg is going to fall off!

- Stand with your feet pointing slightly outward, tailbone tucked under your back. Squeeze your buttocks muscles as tightly and for as long as you can. Hold until muscle failure. Repeat periodically until the

pain is gone.

Lower Back

Six-Inch Straight Leg Raise

This exercise should relieve leg and lower

back pain. The exercise will wear out your gluteal

and psoas muscles. Your psoas muscles are the

primary connectors between your torso and your

legs. They affect your posture and help to stabilize

your spine.

Do not lift your head while attempting this

exercise. You do not want to wear out your upper

abdominal muscles before the job is done. While

lying in the supine position (flat on your back), with

your palms down and hands under your buttocks,

extend the legs straight out.

Resolving Pain

1. Raise your feet six inches off the ground or a flat surface, with your legs fully extended. At the same time, tighten your gluteal muscles as tightly as possible and hold until you achieve muscle failure.

2. You may also place a large book or other object on your stomach. This ensures that your back remains flat while doing the exercise. Make sure the object is not too heavy.

Buttock Exercise to Decrease Resting Tone
Exercise One

When in bed at nighttime, in the supine position, hold your buttocks as tightly as you can, then release, so you're "on," holding your buttocks as tight and as long as you can, then "off." Continue until you fall asleep.

Exercise Two

For this exercise, *do not* put your weight on a sock that is hard enough to cause you excruciating pain. This will make your pain worse. Stop if you get a muscle cramp. This exercise teaches the muscle not to be so tight, so that you will not feel tenderness when you prop yourself on the sock, which acts a fulcrum or pivot point of your body for the exercise.

1. Stand with your buttocks clenched tightly, pushing your legs to the outside to tense up the quads and the outer quads. Repeat until you have muscle failure.

2. Put a wadded sock as a fulcrum on the floor. Drape your body over the sock and put weight on the sock. Check the area that acts like the rotator cuff of the hip, on the outside and back where the leg comes into the pelvis. When you feel the tender spot, hold you buttocks as tight as you can, as long as you can, until you can relax and not feel the tenderness in the area.

Leaning on Shins and Knees

While kneeling on shins and knees with your shoulders back and pelvis forward, lean back engaging the muscles in the area of pain. Hold this position.

Leg Lifts

1. Lie down on your back and put your hands palms down, under your buttocks.

2. Hold your buttocks tightly and raise your leg six inches.

3. Hold your leg in this position until you have muscle failure. Your leg might actually begin to shake.

Taking the muscle to its failure point means it can't be tense anymore, so you'll stop hurting. Your pain may not stop on the very first try, because you have a buildup of lactic acid that needs to be released from your body.

Resolving Pain

Knees

Seated Straight Leg Raise/Tensing Quads

1. While seated in a chair, pull your toes toward your nose, with your knee in a locked position.

2. Slowly lift the leg and hold it up as high as it will go.

3. Then gently lower it down twelve inches and hold it in that position for several seconds.

4. Elevate slowly to the fully extended raised position and hold it again for several seconds.

5. Continue this exercise until fatigued.

One Leg Standing Heel Rise Exercise

The objective of this exercise is to push yourself to the edge by seeing how much knee bend you can hold while doing the heel exercise. DO NOT do anything that causes significant pain. A little discomfort is okay. Pain is not.

1. Standing next to a counter with fingertips on the counter, but not leaning on the counter, lift one foot and stand on a straight leg.

2. Raise your heel so that you're standing on the ball of your foot.

3. Slowly drop back to the flatfooted position.

4. If this caused no significant knee discomfort, then bend your knee slightly and

hold while you perform a heel rise again on the same foot.

5. Gradually working to hold your knee in a more bent position while performing the heel rise repeatedly. Do this exercise slowly to see how much knee bend you can hold while doing the heel raise without hurting your knee.

Imagery

For any of this to work, your body needs to be relaxed. This is why imagery is so important. It can help you let go and relax. Sometimes you have to visualize what you're trying to get your body to do before you can do it.

Say Ahh . . .

Close your eyes and imagine you have a helium balloon connected to your head that keeps it upright. Then, release your logical thinking. Move your thinking focus to your center, which is located in the middle of your sternum. When you get your mind to your center, release your breath and say, "Ahh." This is a habit you need to get into. You're retraining your body. You're releasing the tensions, concerns and annoyances of life. This will allow you to view the world very differently.

Think from Your Center

Allowing your thoughts to come from your center rather than your analytical brain will help you relax and accept situations as they are, rather than fretting over what you can't change. If you're a *thinker* type your brain can work against you.

To train yourself to think from your center, close your eyes and visualize your center. Take several deep breaths in and out. Open your eyes and focus on something from that feeling of being centered. Think from your center means you let go of judgment, angst and trying to control the world around you. Just let things be.

Practice, as you walk around doing what you do—viewing life and situations, accepting things as they are. Is someone at work particularly bothersome? Think about them from your center, rather than your brain. If they're annoying you on a particular day, let it go. Tell yourself to stop being frustrated. The situation is what it is. The person is who they are. Fretting over your frustration will not help you, the other person or the situation.

Summary

The techniques described in this chapter will help you use your hand or piriformis muscle to assess whether the self-protection mechanism is engaged. You need to do this repeatedly to keep your pain away. It should become a part of your daily routine.

Whatever you do, if you experience more pain or excruciating pain, STOP IMMEDIATELY to keep from injuring yourself worse, or engaging the self-protection mechanism.

All of these techniques are intended to relax your body. Even taking your muscles to muscle failure is intended to release tension. The more

relaxed you are, the better the techniques will work.

Case Studies

Many of my patients have escaped their pain using the philosophy and techniques described in this book. I hope these stories of their successes will encourage you to take action and take the first steps to overcome your pain.

The Car Accident

This is the story of a patient of mine, who came to me nine months after a terrible car accident, telling me she wanted to "get herself back." She came to me because she knew I would treat her injuries and pain holistically.

In the accident, my patient was sitting in the front passenger side of the car on a freeway, where everyone was traveling at least sixty miles per hour. An 18-wheeler clipped a car, which caused it to come right at them. To avoid a head-on collision, the driver barely veered left, so that the oncoming car hit the patient's side of the car. The car the patient was in rolled twice and she was knocked unconscious. She came to briefly, as the car she was in flipped over and was spinning upside down on the pavement, then she blacked out again. It's a miracle that anyone survived the crash. Fortunately, an emergency room tech who was in the car behind them jumped out and pounded on the window, telling my patient not to move.

When the emergency vehicles arrived, they strapped everyone who was in the accident to boards. They spent twelve hours in the emergency room. My patient had some broken bones and a head injury. In the following months, she did many things to try to recover. She worked with a physical therapist, chiropractor; took muscle relaxers and pain medications, steroid injections and still suffered greatly with head, neck and back pain. She saw a neurologist, who had not suggested surgery, but she knew that's probably where they were headed next.

This patient knew my reputation for helping people with these types of injuries, and needed relief from her pain, because it was ruining her life.

This woman had been my patient for fifteen years when she had the car accident. To deal with her injuries, she tried all the traditional methods she could think of first, then knew that she needed a more holistic solution. When she came to me, we spent a week using the relaxation and muscle relaxing exercises that I've outlined in this book.

Her friends and family said that after that week, she

was back to her regular self. She was fifty-one years

old at the time of the accident, and now said she felt

like she was thirty years old again.

What she thought was damage done was

nothing more than pain created by the built-in self-

protection mechanism. Her persistent pain was not

so much from the injuries as her body's reaction to

the injuries.

The Overachiever

Another patient, who I would describe as a

highly active overachiever, was in a car accident

and could not walk for four days. When she was

able to move around, she was afraid to exercise

because the more active she was, the more she hurt.

I told her we needed to get her out of the fear-of-pain cycle and into problem-solver mode. Thinking of herself as a problem-solver would hopefully keep her from playing the victim. I explained that getting over the pain is a dynamic process, because she couldn't just do an exercise once and walk away from it. Also, I reminded her that she could not do anything that caused her to hurt because that would invoke the self-protection mechanism.

She totally agreed that she shouldn't act as a victim, which is good for someone overcoming pain. I reminded her that pain is information and indicates how she might be holding herself too tightly.

Resolving Pain

I explained how if someone hurts, the person has a tendency to guard the body, which she understood. I continued to explain that she was creating a context for her pain by flinching, so that her body and muscles were tensed based on the fear of having pain. I showed her how to find the tender spot on her hand and relax her shoulders to relieve tension and pain.

She told me that getting in the car was still intensely painful. I observed that she had a tendency to dedicate herself to a task, even when it required self-sacrifice. This patient has a problem-solver personality and is competitive by nature, so her mind and body go to "fix it" mode when she even fears hurting. Her self-protection mechanism kicks in aggressively, so it took time for her to tame the response to pain. The first step for her was to be conscious of tensing up, then training herself to relax on an ongoing basis.

We discussed further how she couldn't *make* herself relax. She needed to *allow* herself to relax. I told her it would take more effort in the beginning to break her body's pattern of tensing up. I explained the connection between losing her pain and having peace of mind. In our conversation, she realized she had to literally change her mindset from trying to control and fix everything to letting go and relaxing.

When she asked about returning to the gym to work out, I told her to be hyper-vigilant to any pain she felt. I showed her how pain at one point in her body is connected to other parts of the body. It's not just one place that is impacted, but a whole system of things.

Then I showed her the technique for dismantling the self-protection mechanism. Within a few weeks, she saw results because she worked consistently and diligently to apply these techniques.

The Sports Injury

One of my patients was playing basketball when someone hit him on the left side of his neck with an elbow. It hurt quite a bit at first in the shoulder and neck. In about ten seconds, it started to ease, and he felt better. He decided it was fine and that it didn't bother him that much. He thought it was just a bruise, so he finished out the game. The next day he went back to the gym to play basketball. When he went up to block a shot his whole shoulder, back and neck on the left side got really tight. Then his shoulder had a needle-type pain. The next morning when he woke up, he was in so much pain he could not go to work.

In this case, the tissue damage initially caused his pain. The predictable response was more pain. To help this patient, I first had to help him manage the pain due to flinching, then figure out how to deal with the pain that remained due to the initial injury. I helped him dismantle his self-protection mechanism by having him lie on his side, taking a deep breath, letting it go and dropping his shoulders "to the floor." We repeated this several times.

Resolving Pain

My associate and I helped him with a few more exercises and ultimately he got the total relief he needed, without any further treatments or interventions.

Plantar Fasciitis

The plantar fascia is a wide flat tendon that attaches from the front of the heel to the ball of the foot. The plantar fascia acts like a shock-absorbing bowstring, supporting the arch of your foot.

My patient wondered out loud why his heel hurt after driving to and from work. I explained that the traffic and all the intense focusing he needed to do caused his buttocks to tense up, which actually causes the problem with plantar fasciitis. The more he flinches his glutes and pulls his legs in to avoid pain from the foot that hurts, the worse the problem gets.

To figure out how to relieve his pain, we had to first determine how to deal with the excess tone in his buttocks. To help him understand how things work, I demonstrated how pain in his foot was actually connected to that whole side of his body. As he relaxed his buttocks, the plantar fascia relaxed, relieving his pain. Now he understood the system of pain in his body.

To help this patient, I had him lie on his side and pull his knees to his chest. He was resting on his piriformis, and it was predictably tender. I explained that his leg would pull up into his buttocks anticipating pain in the foot, just like he would pull his hand away from the flame in a hot fire. The buttocks are the most stubborn part of the body, so it's a more difficult place to dismantle the self-protection mechanism. When it feels attacked, it's going to do everything it can to protect him.

I also prescribed potassium to relieve him of cramping. That way he would be able to hold his glutes tightly enough and long enough to take them to muscle failure. At muscle failure, his muscles would release tension due to fatigue.

This is an example of a patient who is physically and spiritually strong, so fatiguing the muscles was a little harder for him than it would be for others. He walked out of the office with no pain and continued doing the exercises so the pain wouldn't return.

Shot Knees

I had a patient who was a flight attendant, complaining of horrible knee pain. The X-rays I took of her knees confirmed severe degenerative changes, with narrowing of joint spaces.

We knew that eventually she would need a knee replacement surgery. In the meantime, I gave her some exercises to relieve her pain. After fifteen minutes of treatment using some of the techniques described in this book, she was able to walk around with no pain.

She was so happy that she started sobbing and exclaimed, "I can't believe I have no pain! At this moment I have no pain at all."

Carpal Tunnel

The carpal tunnel is a narrow tunnel located between your wrist and hand that has a floor of

small carpal bones and ceiling of flexor
retinaculum, which the ulnar nerves pass through.
This nerve includes motor neurons for strength and
sensory neurons for feeling. The nerves are
compressed at the carpal tunnel, so when the nerve
becomes severely inflamed and swells, it may not
fit through the tunnel properly. This condition may
be caused by a number of things, including arthritis
or repeated movements that inflame the nerves.

One of my patients is a middle-aged
commercial truck driver, who drives cross- country
in an 18-wheeler. When he is not shifting gears, he
drives with his right hand. He was losing his grip
and strength on the steering wheel and experiencing
pain and numbness. He had carpal tunnel syndrome

in only one of his hands, but we had to get his entire body to relax in order to deal with the issue.

On his first visit, I used manipulation to open up the tunnel to begin relieving the pain and inflammation. This patient had excessive tone in his muscles, so getting them to relax took several weeks. His condition developed over several months, but after a few weeks using the manipulation techniques, he experienced complete relief in his hand.

Tennis Elbow

Tennis elbow is a condition where the outer part of the elbow becomes painful and tender. The problem can extend to the back of the forearm and also weaken grip strength. Typically, this is initially caused by overuse of the muscles in the back of the forearm, commonly caused by aggressively swinging at a tennis ball too late to connect. People with this condition are often trying to muscle the ball rather than use the body's torque to hit a powerful shot. This same type of problem occurs with golfers, racquetball and baseball/softball players.

I had a patient who started to feel discomfort associated with tennis elbow. She did not hurt that badly, so she continued to play without treatment. By continuing to play through the pain for several weeks, my patient created a context for the pain by engaging the self-protection mechanism. I did some manipulation techniques with her that simulated what a tennis elbow strap would do. This helps stop the pain initially, so we can counteract the context for the pain, which was created by continuing to play in spite of it. I taught her some of the biofeedback techniques described in this book. I convinced her not to play through her pain, rather to disengage her flinching reflex and relax. Using biofeedback and stopping the context for her pain, she felt much better after a few weeks.

Summary

In looking at patient conditions, I always need to see if they're creating a context for pain by engaging the self-protection mechanism. While I'm always going to find out about the initial pain that could have been caused by tissue damage, most likely the biggest part of the patient's issue is from flinching in fear of more pain.

Pain is rarely localized to the patient's initial complaint. My patient who had plantar fasciitis had a starting point for pain way above his foot. In his case, the stress of driving in traffic did not help matters. That stress caused his muscles to tense, and the fear of pain in the foot caused him to draw his foot and leg into his body.

During the many years I've been practicing, looking at patient conditions from a holistic perspective has allowed me to help many of them get relief. The body has an amazing power to heal itself when we give it the right conditions. Just remember that when you have pain, your body is trying to communicate something to you, and it's information you can use to help you get relief.

Resolving Pain

Your Pain-Free Life!

I am so grateful that I have a solution for people who are in chronic pain. As I have said before, there is no reason to go around all wadded up, and in chronic pain. The methods I've outlined here will help you figure out if you're flinching, so you can focus on the areas you need to relax. Your pain-free life requires vigilance and consistent effort to change the way you live in your body.

Interestingly, people who are driven to succeed often struggle to use these techniques well because they try to *make* themselves get better. The fact is *acceptance* is a key for these techniques to work. And when I say acceptance, I don't mean that they accept that they have to live with the pain. I mean acceptance that leads to peace of mind, acceptance that it's okay to relax. Acceptance that using these techniques and the process consistently will produce results. When you're dismantling your self-protection mechanism and taking your muscles to fatigue, you won't be successful if you become impatient with the process.

Viewing the world from your center instead of your brain leads to acceptance of the world around you. Your mantra can become "it is what it is." Do you feel constant conflict with someone at work? Don't let that person control you or your behavior. Let them deal with their own problems. You cannot change how they act. All you can change is what you do, how you respond and the internal emotions and thoughts you have regarding that person.

Attitude, anxiety and depression are projections of dynamic thinking. Some think of the future, or what could happen. You can create fear of the future and live in anxiety, or you can develop an attitude of appreciation.

You can approach it this way. "This is my life; I can choose where to focus the camera and the picture I see through the lens. I'm the only one who controls it."

Direct your camera and focus it toward what is beautiful, hopeful and gives you inner peace. When you choose an attitude that is non-judgmental, grateful and positive, you'll be comfortable in your own skin. You can see the world clearly and think from your center.

Resolving Pain

Even though the pain from my fall and the ten years of suffering were not pleasant, if that had not happened to me, I might not have discovered these effective techniques that I learned and now use with my patients. It is my sincerest hope that you'll find relief in your journey to a pain-free life, and I hope reading this book was your first step.